Mediterranean Smoothies, Soups & Much More

Need New Recipes? Have a Look to These New Mediterranean Cookbook

Mateo Buscema

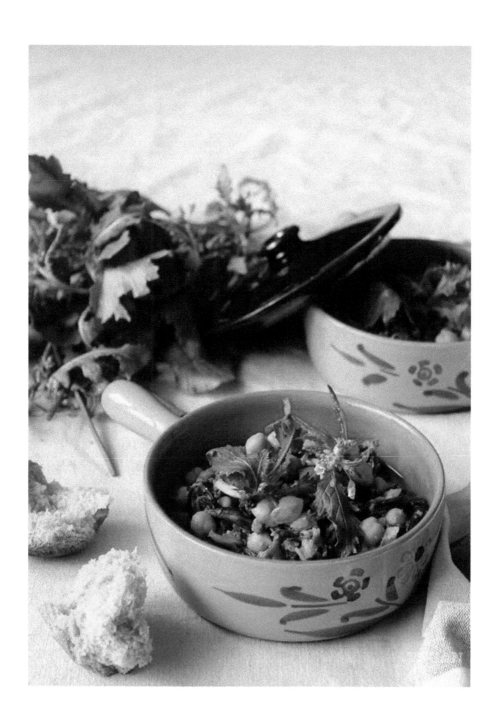

TABLE OF CONTENTS

Red pepper and walnut dip

Ingredients

- 2 teaspoon of cumin powder
- 1 clove of garlic
- The juice of half a lemon
- 2/3 cup of chopped walnuts
- ¼ teaspoon of cayenne powder
- 1 cup of chopped roasted red bell peppers
- 4 tablespoons of tomato paste
- 2 tablespoons of extra virgin olive oil
- ¼ cup of rolled oats

Directions

1. Place all the ingredients in a food processor.
2. Blend until smooth.
3. Serve and enjoy.

Simple Italian minestrone soup

The Italian minestrone soup is perfectly brimmed with variety of vegetables, pasta, and beans.

The thick flavorful tomato broth with some rosemary and herbs gives this soup a total draw.

Ingredients

- 1 small yellow onion chopped
- 2 celery stalks diced
- Salt and pepper
- Large handful chopped parsley
- 2 carrots chopped
- 1pinch Parmesan cheese rind optional
- 1/4 cup of extra virgin olive oil
- 6 cups of broth vegetable or chicken broth
- 1 15 ounces can kidney beans
- 4 garlic cloves minced
- 1 cup green beans fresh
- ½ teaspoon of rosemary
- Grated Parmesan cheese to serve (optional)
- 1 15 ounces of can crushed tomatoes
- 1 teaspoon of paprika
- 2 – 3 springs fresh thyme

- Handful fresh basil leaves
- 1 zucchini or dices yellow squash
- 1 bay leaf
- 2 cups of cooked small pasta

Directions

1. In a large oven, heat the extra virgin olive oil over medium heat until shimmering without smoke.
2. Add carrots, onions, and celery.
3. Increase the heat to medium-high let cook while tossing regularly until the veggies soften somehow for 5 minutes.
4. Add the garlic continue to cook for more 5 minutes, keep tossing.
5. Add the zucchini or yellow squash and green beans the content.
6. Season with rosemary, paprika, and a generous pinch of kosher salt and pepper, then toss to combine.
7. Add the broth, crushed tomatoes, bay leaf, fresh thyme, and Parmesan rind.
8. Boil, then reduce the heat to let simmer for 20 minutes covering the pot partially.
9. Uncover the pot to add the kidney beans let cook for 5 – 10 minutes.
10. Stir in the parsley and fresh basil at once.

11. Stir in the cooked pasta and simmer briefly till the pasta is warmed through, if you want to serve immediately. Ensure not to overcook.

12. Remove the cheese rind and bay leaf.

13. Taste and adjust seasoning accordingly to your taste.

14. Serve the minestrone when hot in dinner bowls and then sprinkle with grated Parmesan which is optional.

15. Enjoy

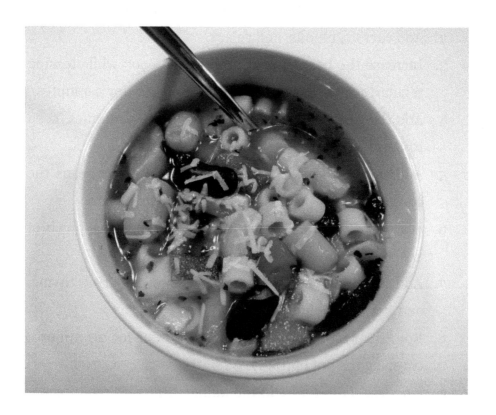

Tomato gazpacho soup

Tomato gazpacho soup blends variety of fresh vegetables with flavorful appetizers.

Garlic and onion gives this recipe the desired taste and aroma.

Ingredients

- 1 cucumber
- 1/4 cup of water
- 2 tablespoon of extra virgin olive oil
- 1 small onion
- A pinch of black pepper
- 1 green pepper
- 2 small slices of sourdough bread
- 1 garlic clove
- 2 tablespoon of apple vinegar
- 2.2 pounds of ripe tomatoes
- 1/4 tablespoon of salt

Directions

1. Boil water in a pot.
2. Place tomatoes the boiling water till the skin starts coming off.

3. Remove the tomatoes let them cool down.
4. Peel off the softened tomato skin and dice.
5. Combine and place vegetables and bread in the blender.
6. Blend until all ingredients until smooth.
7. Taste and adjust accordingly.
8. Serve and enjoy with a drizzle of oil.

5-ingredients spring vegetable soup

This spring vegetable is readily available all year round.

It is light, purely vegetarian for a perfect Mediterranean Sea diet with vitamin boosting properties.

Ingredients

- 1 vegetable stock cube
- 2 tablespoon of sunflower oil
- 2 large potatoes
- 3 medium carrots
- 1 cup of frozen
- 3 celery stalks
- 1 small onion
- Salt

Directions

1. Dice your onion peeled.
2. Sauté for 4 minutes while stirring infrequently over medium heat.

3. Add sliced carrots, celery, potatoes as well as peas to a pot.
4. Sauté for briefly, then add 1.5 liter of water.
5. Season with salt.
6. Bring to boil.
7. Place in vegetable stock cube over reduced heat.
8. Cook for 30 minutes.
9. Serve and enjoy.

Greek avgolemono soup

This recipe is a lemon flavored egg made into a soup with broth and it is highly fragrant and silky.

Ingredients

- 2 large eggs
- ½ cup of finely chopped carrots
- ½ cup of finely chopped celery
- 2 garlic cloves, finely chopped
- 2 bay leaves
- 1 cup of rice
- ½ cup of finely chopped green onions
- Extra virgin olive oil
- Fresh parsley for garnish
- 8 cups of low-sodium chicken broth
- Salt and pepper
- 2 cooked boneless chicken breast pieces, shredded
- ½ cup of freshly-squeezed lemon juice

Directions

1. Start by heating 1 tablespoon of olive oil on medium-high heat until shimmering without smoke in a large oven.

2. Add the celery, carrots, and green onions, toss together.

3. Sauté briefly and stir in the garlic.

4. Add the chicken broth and bay leaves, immediately increase the heat to high.

5. After the liquid is at a rolling boil, add the rice together with the salt and pepper.

6. Lower the heat to medium-low let simmer for 20 minutes.

7. Stir in the cooked chicken.

8. In another separate medium mixing dish, whisk the lemon juice with the eggs.

9. Add 2 ladles-full of the broth as you whisk.

10. Add the sauce to the chicken soup when it is fully combined, make sure to stir.

11. Immediately, remove from heat source.

12. Use the fresh parsley for garnishing, if you desire.

13. Serve and enjoy with bread.

Chunky vegan lentil soup

This recipe entails variety of vegetables and warm spices along with fresh herbs.

It is a wonderful one pot Mediterranean Sea diet salad.

Ingredients

- Extra virgin olive oil
- 2 celery stalks, chopped
- 1 cup of chopped fresh parsley, stems removed
- ½ teaspoon of ground cinnamon
- 1 russet potato, small diced
- 1 ½ cups of green lentils
- 4 garlic cloves, chopped
- 1 zucchini squash, diced
- 2 tablespoons of fresh lime or lemon juice
- 1 medium yellow onion, chopped
- Salt and pepper
- 1 teaspoon of ground coriander
- Bread to serve
- 1 bulk carrot, chopped
- 1 teaspoon of ground cumin
- 1 teaspoon of turmeric powder
- ½ teaspoon of cayenne pepper

- 3 cups of canned diced tomatoes with juice
- 2 ½ cup of water
- lime or lemon wedges to serve

Directions

1. Place the lentils in a bowl and cover with water.
2. Wash and soak for 10 minutes. Drain well.
3. In a large heavy pot, heat 2 tablespoons of extra virgin olive oil.
4. Add onions, carrot, celery, and potatoes let cook over medium-high heat for 5 minutes, stirring regularly.
5. Add garlic and zucchini. Cook for another 5 minutes, stirring regularly.
6. Add lentils, salt and pepper and spices.
7. Toss to combine, then add the tomatoes and water.
8. Bring everything to a boil for 5 minutes.
9. Lower the heat cover and let simmer for 20 minutes.
10. Remove from heat and stir in parsley and lime juice.
11. Transfer to serving bowls and top with a drizzle of extra virgin olive oil .
12. Serve and enjoy hot with crusty bread.

Mediterranean spicy spinach lentil soup

Ingredients

- 1 large yellow onion, finely chopped
- • 1 ½ teaspoons of ground cumin
- 2 teaspoons of dried mint flakes
- Pinch of sugar
- 1 tablespoon of flour
- 6 cups of low-sodium vegetable broth
- 2 cups of chopped flat leaf parsley
- 1 ½ teaspoons of sumac
- Private reserve Greek extra virgin olive oil
- 1 large garlic clove, chopped
- 1 ½ teaspoons of crushed red peppers
- 3 cups of water, more if needed
- 12 ounces of frozen cut leaf spinach
- 1 ½ teaspoons of ground coriander
- Salt and pepper
- 1 ½ cups of green lentils or small brown lentils, rinsed
- 1 lime, juice of lemon

Directions

1. In a large ceramic pot, heat 2 tablespoons of olive oil.
2. Add the chopped onions and Sauté until golden brown.
3. Add the garlic, all the spices, dried mint, sugar, and flour.
4. Let cook for 2 minutes on medium heat stirring regularly.
5. Add the broth and water.
6. Increase the heat to high and boil to a rolling point.
7. Add the frozen spinach and the lentils.
8. Continue to cook for 5 minutes on high heat.
9. Lower the heat and let simmer when covered for 20 minutes.
10. Once the lentils are fully cooked, stir in the lime juice and chopped parsley.
11. Remove from the heat source and let settle covered for 5 minutes.
12. Serve and enjoy hot with pita bread.

Greek red lentil soup

Trust me, this is a huge surprise to your taste buds.

Flavored with onions and garlic and sweetness of the sweet carrots with tomatoes infused with cumin, oregano and rosemary makes this a perfect Mediterranean Sea diet.

Ingredients

- 1 large onion, chopped
- 3 teaspoons of dry oregano
- 1 ½ teaspoons of cumin
- 1 teaspoon of rosemary
- Juice of 2 lemons
- Fresh parsley for garnish
- ½ teaspoon of red pepper flakes
- Extra virgin olive oil
- 2 dry bay leaves
- Crumbled feta cheese to serve
- 7 cups of low-sodium vegetable broth
- 3 garlic cloves, minced
- 2 carrots, chopped
- 2 cups of red lentils , rinsed and drained
- Kosher salt
- 1 cup of crushed tomatoes

- Zest of 1 lemon

Directions

1. Heat 3 tablespoons of extra virgin olive oil until shimmering without smoke.
2. Add onions, carrots and garlic let cook for 4 minutes, stirring regularly.
3. Add spices and bay leaves.
4. Cook for a few seconds till fragrant, keep stirring.
5. Add crushed tomatoes together with the broth, and lentils.
6. Season with kosher salt and boil.
7. Reduce the heat let simmer for 20 minutes.
8. Remove from heat, let cool then immerse blender to puree.
9. Return soup to heat, and stir to warm through.
10. Add lemon zest, lemon juice, and fresh parsley.
11. Move soup to serving bowls and top with extra virgin olive oil.
12. Serve and enjoy.

Roasted tomato basil soup

This Mediterranean Sea diet recipe combines aromatic fresh herbs and warm spices.

The extra virgin olive oil will give your taste buds the final blast.

Ingredients

- Extra virgin olive oil
- 2 teaspoons of thyme leaves
- 2 medium yellow onions chopped
- Splash of lime juice
- 5 garlic cloves minced
- Salt and pepper
- 1 cup of canned crushed tomatoes
- 3 lb.. Roma tomatoes halved
- 2 ½ cups of water
- 3 carrots peeled and cut into small chunks
- ½ teaspoon of ground cumin
- 2 ounces of fresh basil leaves
- 4 fresh thyme springs
- 1 teaspoon of dry oregano
- ½ teaspoon of paprika

Directions

1. Heat your oven to 450°F.
2. In a large mixing bowl, combine tomatoes and carrot pieces.
3. Add a drizzle of extra virgin olive oil, and season with kosher salt and black pepper. Toss.
4. Transfer to a large baking sheet and spread well in one layer.
5. Roast in heated oven for about 30 minutes.
6. Let cool for 10 minutes when ready.
7. Transfer the roasted tomatoes and carrots to the large bowl of a food processor fitted with a blade.
8. Add just a tiny bit of water and blend.
9. In a large cooking pot, heat 2 tablespoons of extra virgin olive oil over medium heat until shimmering without smoke.
10. Add onions let cook for 3 minutes.
11. Add garlic and cook briefly until golden.
12. Pour the roasted tomato mixture into the cooking pot.
13. Stir in crushed tomatoes with water, basil, thyme, and spices.
14. Season with a little kosher salt and black pepper.
15. Boil, then reduce the heat and cover part-way.
16. Let simmer for 20 minutes.
17. Remove the thyme springs and transfer tomato basil soup to serving bowls.

18. Serve and enjoy with lime juice if you desire.

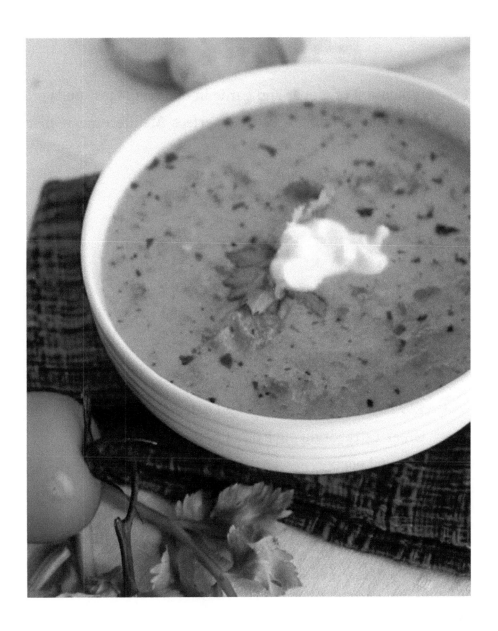

Creamy roasted carrot soup with ginger

The combination of ginger and garlic in one recipe just pulls off the flavor side of it making it a perfect Mediterranean diet recipe.

It is gluten free.

Ingredients

- 1 teaspoon of ground coriander
- 3 lb. carrots peeled
- 1 teaspoon of allspice
- Fresh mint
- 1 ½ cup unsweetened half and half
- Greek extra virgin olive oil
- Salt and pepper
- 1 teaspoon of grated fresh ginger
- 5 ½ cups low-sodium vegetable broth divided
- 4 garlic cloves chopped

Directions

1. Preheat your oven ready to 425°F.

2. Organize the carrots on a large lightly oiled sheet pan.

3. Season lightly with salt and pepper and drizzle generously with olive oil.

4. Roast in the oven for 45 minutes, turn over mid-way through.

5. When the carrots are ready, set aside briefly.

6. Cut the carrots into chunks and place them in a large food processor with the garlic, ginger and broth.

7. Puree until the mixture is smooth.

8. Transfer the carrot puree to a heavy cooking pot.

9. Add the remaining broth, coriander and allspice.

10. Place the pot on medium heat let boil as you watch. Stir occasionally.

11. Reduce the heat to low, stir in the heavy cream to heat through.

12. Transfer to serving bowls and garnish with fresh mint leaves.

13. Serve and enjoy with rustic bread.

Mediterranean bean soup recipe with tomato pesto

Ingredients

- 1 Large russet potato, peeled, diced
- 2 cups of cooked chickpeas
- 1 15-oz. can of diced tomatoes
- ½ cup grated Parmesan cheese
- 1 tablespoon of ground coriander
- 1 teaspoon of Spanish paprika
- 5 cups of low sodium vegetable broth
- 8-oz. of frozen spinach, no need to thaw
- 2 cups of cooked red kidney beans
- 1 tablespoon of white vinegar
- Basil leaves
- ⅓ cup of toasted pine nuts for garnish
- 1 medium yellow onion, chopped
- Salt and pepper
- 3 large garlic cloves
- Greek extra virgin olive oil
- 2 cups of cooked cannellini beans
- 1 ½ cup of diced fresh tomatoes
- 15 large basil leaves

Directions

1. In a large oven, heat 2 tablespoons of olive oil.
2. Add the diced potatoes and onions over low heat and let cook for 5 minutes, toss.
3. Add tomatoes, vinegar, spices, salt and pepper. Stir.
4. Continue to cook for 4 minutes.
5. Add vegetable broth with frozen spinach.
6. Increase the heat to medium boil for 4 minutes.
7. Add the kidney beans together with the cannellini beans, and chickpeas.
8. Boil again, then reduce heat to low let cook for 20 minutes.
9. In the bowl of a food processor, place garlic and tomatoes.
10. Blend briefly to combine.
11. Add basil and puree.
12. Drizzle in the olive oil a little bit at a time as the processor is still running.
13. Transfer the thick tomato pesto to a bowl, and stir in grated Parmesan.
14. Stir in the tomato pesto when soup is ready.
15. Transfer to serving bowl then top each bowl with a few basil leaves and toasted pine nuts.
16. Serve and enjoy with crusty bread.

Mushroom barley soup

Ingredients

- 1 cup of pearl barley rinsed
- Kosher salt
- 1 yellow onion, chopped
- 6 cups of low-sodium broth
- ½ cup of packed chopped parsley
- 2 celery stalks, chopped
- 1 carrot, chopped
- 8 oz.. of white mushrooms, cleaned and chopped
- ½ cup of canned crushed tomatoes
- Black pepper
- 1 teaspoon of coriander
- 4 garlic cloves, chopped
- Extra virgin olive oil
- ½ teaspoon of to 3/4 teaspoon of smoked paprika
- 16 oz. of baby Bella mushrooms
- ½ teaspoon of cumin

Directions

1. In a large Oven, heat extra virgin olive oil over medium heat until shimmering without smoke.

2. Add baby bell mushrooms let cook until mushrooms are soft.

3. Remove from the pot, keep for later.

4. In the same pot, add a little more extra virgin olive oil.

5. Add onions together with the garlic, carrots, celery, and chopped white mushrooms.

6. Cook for 5 minutes over medium-high heat.

7. Then, season with salt and pepper.

8. Add the crushed tomatoes and spices let cook for 3 minutes, toss regularly.

9. Add broth and pearl barley give it a rolling boil for 5 minutes.

10. Lower the heat and let simmer over low heat for 45 minutes until the barley is tender.

11. Add the cooked Bella mushrooms back to the pot and stir to combine.

12. Continue to cook for 5 minutes.

13. Add fresh parsley.

14. Serve and enjoy.

Pressure pot chickpea soup

The chickpea soup is another loaded recipe with variety of vegetables and fresh herbs as well as warm spices.

It is gluten free, low carb yet high plant protein based.

Ingredients

- 1 yellow onion, chopped
- 15 oz. can of chopped tomatoes with juice
- 3 garlic cloves, minced
- Salt
- 6 cups low-sodium vegetable broth
- 2 carrots, chopped
- 1 green bell pepper, cored, chopped
- 1 oz. chopped fresh cilantro
- 4 red chili peppers
- 1 teaspoon of ground coriander
- 1 teaspoon of ground cumin
- 2 cups dry chickpeas
- 1 teaspoon of Aleppo pepper
- 1 lemon, juice of
- ½ teaspoon of ground turmeric
- ½ teaspoon of ground allspice
- Greek extra virgin olive oil

Directions

1. Place chickpeas in a large bowl and add plenty of water and let soak overnight.
2. Preheat your Pressure Pot by selecting the Sauté function and adjust heat to high.
3. Add 2 tablespoon of extra virgin olive oil let heat until shimmering.
4. Add onions together with the garlic and a pinch of salt let cook for 3 minutes, stirring regularly.
5. Add carrots, bell peppers, and spices. Continue to cook for 4 minutes, stir to soften the vegetables.
6. Add drained chickpeas together with the tomatoes, and broth.
7. Lock your Pressure Pot lid in place.
8. Select the pressure cooking setting and set on high.
9. Set the timer to 15 minutes.
10. Allow time to let pressure release naturally when cooked.
11. Unlock and remove the lid.
12. Stir in lemon juice and fresh cilantro.
13. Taste and adjust accordingly.
14. Transfer to serving bowls and drizzle extra virgin olive oil.
15. Serve and enjoy with crusty bread.

Mediterranean bean soup with tomato pesto

Beans are a reliable source of proteins, therefore combined with a variety of vegetables especially tomatoes, it can feed a crowd.

Ingredients

- 1 15-oz. can of diced tomatoes
- 1 tablespoon of white vinegar
- 3 large garlic cloves
- 1 tablespoon of ground coriander
- 1 Large russet potato, peeled, diced into small cubes
- 1 teaspoon of Spanish paprika
- ½ cup of grated Parmesan cheese
- Salt and pepper
- 5 cups of low sodium vegetable broth
- Greek extra virgin olive oil
- 8-oz. of frozen spinach, no need to thaw
- 20 large basil leaves
- 2 cups of cooked red kidney beans
- 1 ½ cup diced fresh tomatoes
- 1 medium yellow onion, chopped
- 2 cups of cooked cannellini beans

- 2 cups of cooked chickpeas
- Basil leaves for garnish
- ⅓ cup of toasted pine nuts for garnish

Directions

1. In a heavy pot, heat 2 teaspoons of olive oil.
2. Reduce heat to medium and add the diced potatoes and onions let cook for 5 minutes, tossing regularly.
3. Add tomatoes together with the vinegar, spices, salt and pepper. Stir to combine.
4. Let cover for 4 minutes.
5. Add vegetable broth and frozen spinach.
6. Increase the heat to medium let boil for 4 minutes.
7. Add the kidney beans, cannellini beans, and chickpeas.
8. Bring back to a boil.
9. Lower the heat cover let cook for 20 minutes.
10. In the bowl of a food processor, place garlic and tomatoes.
11. Pulse briefly to combine.
12. Then, add basil and puree and drizzle in the olive oil a little bit as the processor is still running.
13. Transfer the thick tomato pesto to a bowl, stir in grated Parmesan.
14. Remove from heat source. Stir in the tomato pesto.
15. Shift to the serving bowl.

16. Top each bowl with a few basil leaves and toasted pine nuts.

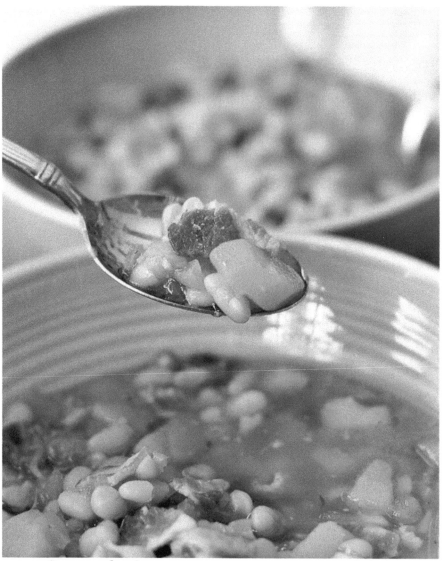

17. Serve and enjoy.

Cream of a roasted cauliflower soup with Mediterranean twist

Ingredients

- 2 teaspoons of ground cumin
- Greek extra virgin olive oil
- 1/4 teaspoon of ground turmeric
- Salt and pepper
- ½ lemon, juice of lemon
- 2 ½ cups of fat-free half and half
- 1 small sweet onion, chopped
- 5 garlic cloves, chopped
- 2 heads of cauliflower, cut into florets
- 1 cup chopped fresh dill
- 2 ½ teaspoon of Sweet Spanish paprika
- 4 cups of low-sodium vegetable broth
- 1 cup of water
- 1 teaspoon of ground sumac

Directions

1. Start by preheating your oven to 425°F.
2. Place cauliflower florets on a large sheet pan.

3. Sprinkle with salt and pepper and drizzle with extra virgin olive oil. Toss.
4. Spread evenly on sheet pan let roast 45 minutes in the oven, make sure to turn midway to balance the sides.
5. In a large heavy pot, heat 2 tablespoons of olive oil until shimmering but without smoke.
6. Add onions and let sauté, over medium heat, until translucent.
7. Add chopped garlic and spices.
8. Stir briefly until fragrant.
9. Add 3/4 the amount of roasted cauliflower.
10. Stir to coat well with the spices, then add vegetable broth and water.
11. Boil, then lower heat to medium.
12. Cover part-way and let simmer for 7 minutes.
13. Remove from heat.
14. Blend cauliflower and liquid until you achieve desired smoothness.
15. Return to a medium heat and stir in the fat-free half and half, and lime juice.
16. Stir in the remainder of roasted cauliflower florets you reserved earlier.
17. Let cook briefly to warm through.
18. Test and adjust salt accordingly.
19. Stir in the chopped dill.
20. Serve and enjoy hot with crusty whole wheat bread.

Curried red lentil and sweet potato soup

Ingredients

- 1 large sweet potato, peeled, cubed
- 1 teaspoon of paprika
- 3 15-oz. cans of vegetable broth
- 1 ½ cup of red lentils, rinsed
- 2 celery ribs, chopped
- 1 large red onion, halved, divided
- 1 teaspoon of mild yellow curry
- Olive oil
- 1 teaspoon of seasoned salt
- 1 bay leaf
- 4 garlic cloves, chopped
- 1 1/4 cup of heavy cream

Directions

1. In a non-stick pan, heat a tablespoon of olive oil.
2. Sauté sliced onions on medium-high until fairly brown and crispy.
3. Remove onions onto a paper towel to drain any excess oil.
4. In a large pot, heat 3 tablespoons of olive oil.

5. Add chopped onions together with the sweet potato and celery let sauté on medium-high for 5 minutes as you stir infrequently.
6. Add garlic, curry, seasoned salt, paprika and bay leaf. Toss toss.
7. Pour in three cans of vegetable broth let cook on medium-high and bring to a boil.
8. As broth is boiling, stir in rinsed red lentils.
9. Let continue to cook for 4 minutes on medium-high heat, stirring occasionally.
10. Lower the heat to medium-low, cover let cook for 7 minutes, stirring occasionally.
11. Test and adjust accordingly.
12. Stir in heavy cream and let cook briefly to warm through.
13. Serve and enjoy with browned and crispy onions.

Easy vegan pumpkin soup

Ingredients

- 2 medium yellow onions, chopped
- ½ teaspoon of organic ground turmeric
- Jalapeno slices for garnish
- 2 garlic cloves, minced
- 1/4 cup pine nuts, toasted in olive oil
- 1 teaspoon of organic ground coriander
- 1 cup of red lentils
- 15 oz. can pumpkin puree
- 3 ½ cups quality vegetable broth
- Salt
- 3 tablespoons of gold raisins
- Extra virgin olive oil
- ½ fresh lemon, juice of
- 1 tablespoon of tomato paste
- 1 Zhoug cilantro pesto
- 1 teaspoon of organic ground cumin

Directions

1. Prepare your Zhoug spicy cilantro paste normally. Keep aside for later.

2. In a heavy pot, heat 2 extra virgin olive oil over medium-high heat until shimmering but without smoke.

3. Add the onions let cook until golden and translucent then toss.

4. Stir in garlic together with the tomato paste, coriander, cumin, and turmeric.

5. Lower heat to medium let cook for 4 minutes, stirring regularly.

6. Add the lentils together with the pumpkin puree, broth and a little salt. Stir.

7. Raise the heat to high let boil for 5 minutes.

8. Then, lower the heat cover only part-way let continue to cook for 20 minutes, stir.

9. Remove from heat let cool briefly.

10. Transfer the lentil pumpkin soup to the bowl of a large food processor blend.

11. Return to pot over medium heat to warm through, stirring occasionally.

12. Stir in raisins together with the fresh lemon juice.

13. Let cook for 4 minutes, stir regularly.

14. Taste adjust accordingly.

15. Divide the lentil pumpkin soup into serving bowls.

16. Then, top with a teaspoon of Zhoug spicy cilantro pesto and toasted pine nuts.

17. Garnish with jalapeno slices, serve.

18. Enjoy.

Herbed vegan potato leek soup

Ingredients

- Salt and pepper
- 6 garlic cloves, peeled
- 1 teaspoon of ground cumin
- 1 cup of fresh cilantro leaves
- 1 teaspoon of sweet paprika
- Greek extra virgin olive oil
- Lemon wedges to serve
- 3 leeks, well-cleaned
- 2 dried bay leaves
- 2 lb. Yukon gold potatoes
- 6 cups of vegetable broth

Directions

1. In a small food processor, blend garlic cloves and fresh cilantro until finely ground into a paste.
2. In a large heavy cooking pot, heat 3 tablespoon of olive oil over medium-high heat until shimmering but with no smoke.
3. Add the garlic and cilantro mixture together with the chopped leeks.
4. Let cook as you toss regularly, until leeks are tender.

5. Add potatoes together with the spices, and a generous dash of salt and pepper. Toss.

6. Add the bay leaves and vegetable broth.

7. Boil for 5 minutes after which lower the to medium and let simmer for another 15 minutes until the potatoes are tender.

8. Turn off heat.

9. Fish the bay leaves out.

10. Using an immersion blender, blend the potato leek to your liking.

11. Place the pot back on stove to heat the soup through over medium heat, stirring.

12. Taste and adjust seasoning accordingly.

13. Transfer soup to serving bowls.

14. Add a generous drizzle of olive oil.

15. Serve with lemon wedges and crusty bread.

16. Enjoy.

Pressure pot stuffed pepper soup

This a true fuss-free recipe using an Pressure pot with two secret ingredients.

It derives its taste from variety of flavors.

Ingredients

- 3 cups of beef broth
- 1 onion
- 2 teaspoons of dried oregano
- 1 pound of lean ground beef
- 1 teaspoon of salt
- 3 garlic cloves, minced
- 1 large green bell pepper
- 1½ cup of roasted peppers , drained
- 2 cups of tomato juice
- 1 tablespoon of sunflower oil
- 2 cups of water
- A pinch of black pepper
- ½ cup of uncooked rice

Directions

1. Turn on the Pressure Pot.

2. Click Sauté then add oil in.

3. Sauté green pepper and onion for 3 minutes

4. Add ground beef and minced garlic.

5. Break up the meat into smaller pieces.

6. Mix.

7. Add roasted peppers and the rest of the ingredients.

8. Mix well, lock the lid in position.

9. Turn the steam valve to sealing.

10. Set time to 5 minutes in the manual and let it run.

11. When the time is up wait for extra 10 minutes.

12. Release the pressure.

13. Taste and season accordingly.

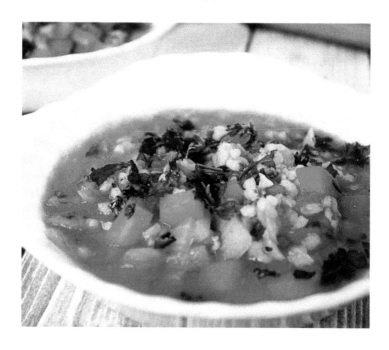

Easy geek lentil soup

This recipe leads to a creamy outcome which, by all means will surprise one's taste buds especially when combined with sweet carrots, onions and garlic.

More so, it is infused with oregano, rosemary, and oregano to increase your lust for it. It is imperative to not that lentils are one of the vital part of a Mediterranean Sea diet and several other legumes.

Ingredients

- 2 dry bay leaves
- 1 teaspoons of rosemary
- 1 ½ teaspoons of cumin
- 1 large chopped onion
- 2 carrots, chopped
- Extra virgin olive oil
- 3 teaspoons of dry oregano
- Crumbled feta cheese
- 1 cup crushed tomatoes
- Fresh parsley for garnish
- 2 cups red lentils , rinsed and drained
- ½ teaspoons of red pepper flakes
- 3 minced garlic cloves

- Zest of 1 lemon
- Juice of 2 lemons
- Kosher salt
- 7 cups low-sodium vegetable broth

Directions

1. Heart about 3 tablespoon of extra virgin oil, endure it does not smoke.
2. Add carrots, garlic, and the onions and cook for 3 – 4 minutes while stirring frequently.
3. Introduce the bay leaves and spices, then while stirring, cook for a few seconds till fragrant.
4. Combine lentils, tomatoes, and the broth and add together, use salt to season.
5. Bring it to boil, reduce the heat to allow it to simmer for 15 – 20 minutes.
6. Reduce the content from the heat source. Cool off and puree in a blender.
7. Pulse until visible cream consistency.
8. Place the soup back on heat, continue to stir to allow even warming.
9. Introduce the lemon juice and parsley.
10. Transfer the soup to serving dishes, of course topped with extra virgin olive oil.
11. Serve with crusty bread of your choice and enjoy.

Easy salmon soup

In just 20 minutes or less, this delicacy of creamy chunks of salmon tucked with incredible flavors typical in the broth with carrots and dill.

The application of lemon juice brings out the taste in this salmon soup.

Ingredients

- 1 teaspoon of dry oregano
- 1 carrot, thinly sliced into rounds
- Zest and juice of 1 lemon
- 4 green onions, chopped
- 3/4 teaspoon of ground coriander
- 4 garlic cloves, minced
- ½ green bell pepper, chopped
- ½ teaspoon of ground cumin
- Kosher salt and black pepper
- 5 cups low-sodium chicken broth
- 1 ounces of fresh dill, divided, chopped
- Extra virgin olive oil
- 1 lb. gold potatoes, thinly sliced into rounds
- 1 lb. salmon skinless fillet, cut into large chunks

Directions

1. In a large pot, heat 2 tablespoons of extra virgin olive oil, allow it to shimmer without smoking.
2. Add the bell pepper, garlic, and onions, cook over medium temperature with constant stirring to produce fragrance in 3 minutes.
3. Introduce ½ of the fresh dill, then stir for 30 minutes.
4. It is time to add the broth, carrots, and potatoes.
5. Add the spices, then season with the kosher salt and black pepper.
6. Boil in a high temperature, reduce the temperature to medium and continue to cook for 5 – 6 minutes.
7. Separately, season the salmon with kosher salt and then introduce it to the pot of soup. Reduce the temperature cook shortly for 3 – 5 minutes to allow the salmon to cook completely.
8. Add and stir in the zest, remaining dill, and lemon juice
9. Transfer your soup to a serving bowl.
10. Serve and enjoy with some crusty breads.

Breakfast egg muffins

These easy to freeze low-carb eggs muffins are a perfect choice of breakfast for anyone who eats eggs.

It is even tastier when serves along with veggies and other salads especially the Mediterranean favorite veggies and salads.

Ingredients

- ½ teaspoon of Spanish paprika
- 1 chopped shallot
- 1 28. 34 g chopped fresh parsley leaves
- 1 small chopped red bell pepper
- 8 large eggs
- 12 cherry tomatoes, halved
- 3 to 4 113 g boneless shredded cooked chicken or turkey
- Salt and Pepper
- Extra virgin olive oil for brushing
- Handful crumbled feta to your liking
- 1/4 teaspoon of ground turmeric (optional)
- 6 to 10 pitted Kalamata olives, chopped

Directions

1. Get a rack, place it in the middle of your oven and start by preheating it to 350°

2. Prepare a muffin pan that can fit 12 muffin cups then brush it all with extra olive oil.

3. Equally divide the tomatoes, shallots, chicken, olives, peppers, extra virgin oil, and parsley.

4. Add the salt, pepper, eggs, and spices in one bowl, then whisk to allow it combine well.

5. Over each of the cups, pour the mixture of eggs, with a small space at the top.

6. Place the muffin pan on top of the sheet pan.

7. Bake it for approximately 25 minutes in a heated oven.

8. Allow it to cool for some time and run some butter along the edges of every muffin.

9. Remove it off the pan

10. Serve and enjoy

Coconut mango overnight oats

This is high energy giving recipe is ideal for families that are quite busy and always on the go. It is fuss free make with mangoes, oats, coconut and other as listed among the ingredients

Ingredients

- 2 teaspoons of shredded coconut
- A pinch of salt
- 2 teaspoons of honey
- ½ cup of diced mango, frozen or fresh
- ½ cup of milk
- 1 teaspoon of chia seeds
- ½ Cup of rolled oats

Directions

1. Start by putting the oats in a jug.
2. Add a pinch of salt.
3. Pour the over milk over the oats in the jar together with all the other ingredients. Blend well.
4. Pack in a closed container and refrigerate overnight.
5. Served chilled and enjoy.

Turmeric hot chocolate

The turmeric hot chocolate has anti-inflammatory properties making a healthier Mediterranean Sea diet choice for anyone.

Ingredients

- 2 teaspoons of honey
- A pinch of cayenne pepper
- 2 teaspoons of coconut oil
- 1 cup of milk
- 1 teaspoon of ground turmeric
- A pinch of black pepper
- 1½ tablespoons of cocoa powder

Directions

1. Firstly, place your milk in a sauce pan.
2. Then, add turmeric, cocoa powder, and coconut oil.
3. Whisk to combine everything.
4. Bring to a boil.
5. Add black pepper and cayenne pepper when the heat is off, stir.
6. Pour in a mug.
7. Allow the mixture to cool.
8. Then add adding honey.
9. Serve and enjoy warm.

Fir tart

Figs fruits are the essential ingredients in making this recipe.

It blends puff pastry and ricotta along with fig filling.

This recipe is perfect for a Mediterranean desert in about 25 minutes.

Ingredients

- 1 puff of pastry sheet, thawed
- 8 ounces of ricotta
- 3 tablespoons of honey
- 12 fresh figs
- 4 tablespoons of almonds, roughly chopped
- 2 teaspoons of shredded coconut

Directions

1. Preheat your oven to 400°F.
2. Mix ricotta together with the honey and figs flesh until well combine in a small dish. Keep for later.
3. Unfold the pastry and roll it out thin.
4. Cut in half.

5. Place all of them onto a baking tray aligned with baking parchment.
6. Cut indentations alongside the edges.
7. Between the two tarts, divide the ricotta mixture and spread over. Make sure the mixture is only in the inner frame cut with the knife.
8. Then cut 2 figs into wedges.
9. Put them on the tart randomly.
10. Then, put the tray in the oven.
11. At 400°F, bake for 12 minutes, the edges should become puffed and the bottom should turn golden brown.
12. Cut each fig into 8 pieces.
13. The almonds should be roughly chopped.
14. Take the tarts out when they are ready.
15. Use the fresh figs for topping, then sprinkle with almonds and coconut.
16. Serve and enjoy warm.

Blueberry turnovers

The recipe combines puff pastry together with homemade blueberry fillings.

This Mediterranean diet is fit for breakfast, lunch or dinner.

Ingredients

- All-purpose flour , for dusting
- ⅓ cup brown sugar
- 1 tablespoon lemon juice
- 1 teaspoon brown sugar
- 1 small egg, beaten
- 2 ounces unsalted butter
- 2 teaspoons cornstarch
- 1 sheet puff pastry, thawed or fresh
- 2 cups frozen blueberries

Directions

1. Combine blueberries, sugar with the lemon juice and simmer for 10 minutes in a small saucepan.
2. Follow by stirring in the butter.
3. Make sure to dilute cornstarch in 1 tablespoon of water in a cup.

4. Add bit of the blueberry sauce, stir well to mix.

5. Pour the cornstarch into the saucepan, make sure to stir until the sauce is thick.

6. Pour it into a bowl when ready, let cool for 30 minutes.

7. Preheat an oven to 400°F.

8. Unfold the puff pastry and roll it out.

9. Cut into squares.

10. Scoop 2 heaped teaspoons blueberry filling in the middle of pastry squares.

11. Run your finger alongside the sides of each square after dipping your finger in water.

12. Lift one tip of the pastry and fold it over the filling towards the opposite tip forming a triangle.

13. To seal, press down the edges.

14. Double-seal with a fork.

15. Place turnovers onto a baking tray.

16. Pierce each turnover to allow steam to escape.

17. Brush with egg wash and sprinkle with brown sugar.

18. Bake in the oven for 15 minutes.

19. When ready, serve and enjoy.

Strawberry coconut tart

This recipe uses simple and easy to find ingredients.

It is quite easy to make from scratch in 35 minutes.

Ingredients

- 2/3 cups of unsweetened desiccated coconut
- 1 stick unsalted butter , melted
- 4 tablespoons of strawberry jam
- 3 tablespoons of powdered sugar
- 1 cup of all-purpose flour
- ½ cup of powdered sugar
- 1 egg white, from a large egg

Directions

1. In a mixing bowl, combine flour with powdered sugar.
2. Add melted butter.
3. Make sure to mix thoroughly with a large spoon.
4. Mix your hands when it begins to form dough.
5. Wrap it and let chill for 30 minutes.
6. Remove it from the fridge and fill the bottom and sides of a pie pan with it. Do not roll.

7. Take a piece of the pastry and press it down. This should be piece by piece until you use up all of it.
8. Spread jam over the crust. Keep aside.
9. Whip the egg white until soft peaks appear.
10. Add sifted sugar and beat until smooth.
11. Stir in the coconut.
12. Pour this mixture over the jam and spread evenly round.
13. Bake in a preheated oven at 350°F for 25-30 minutes.
14. Remove out when ready and let it cool totally.
15. Serve and enjoy.

Traditional Greek salad

Ingredients

- 1 English cucumber partially peeled making a striped pattern
- ½ teaspoon of dried oregano
- Blocks of Greek feta cheese do not crumble the feta, leave it in large pieces
- Greek pitted Kalamata olives a handful to your liking
- 4 teaspoon of quality extra virgin olive oil
- 1 medium red onion
- kosher salt a pinch
- 4 Medium juicy tomatoes
- 1-2 teaspoon of red wine vinegar
- 1 green bell pepper cored

Instruction

1. Begin by cutting the red onions into halves, then slice into crescent moon shape.
2. Cut the tomatoes into wedges or even you can slice others in rounds.
3. Cut the cucumber into half and slice into halves.
4. The bell pepper should be sliced into rings.

5. Combine all the ingredients in the above steps in a large salad dish.

6. Add some pitted Kalamata olives.

7. Using kosher salt, season lightly with some dried oregano.

8. Pour wine vinegar and olive oil all over the salad.

9. Toss gently to combine and blend. Be sure not to over mix.

10. Introduce the feta block right on top and sprinkle with more of the dried oregano.

11. S

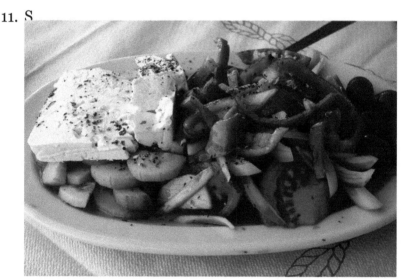

crusty bread and enjoy.

Mediterranean watermelon salad

Watermelon a special healthy gift to the kidney can be used to make a perfect salad using only three main ingredients typically watermelon, feta cheese, cucumber.

Adding fresh mint, honey vinaigrette, and basil propels this recipe to a whole new horizon.

Ingredients

- ½ peeled watermelon cut in cubes
- ½ cup of crumble feta cheese
- 15 fresh chopped mint leaves
- 15 chopped fresh basil leaves
- 1 cucumber
- 2 teaspoon of extra virgin olive oil
- 2 tablespoons of honey
- 2 teaspoons of lime juice
- Pinch of salt

Directions

1. Whisk the honey together with olive oil, pinch of salt, and lime juice.
2. Keep the mixture aside for a while.
3. In a large bowl, serve the platter with sides.
4. Combine the cucumber, fresh herbs, and watermelon together.
5. Top the salad with honey vinaigrette and toss to allow massive combination.
6. Top with feta cheese
7. Sever and enjoy.

Mediterranean chickpea salad

Ingredients

- 1 large thinly sliced eggplant
- Salt
- oil for frying
- 1 cup cooked or canned chickpeas
- 3 tablespoons of Za'atar spice , divided
- 3 Roma tomatoes, diced
- ½ diced English cucumber, diced
- 1 small red onion, sliced in ½ moons
- 1 cup chopped parsley
- 1 cup chopped dill
- 1-2 garlic cloves, minced
- 1 large lime, juice of
- ⅓ cup Early Harvest extra virgin olive oil
- Salt and Pepper

Directions

1. Place the eggplants on a tray large enough to accommodate them, then sprinkle with salt.
2. Allow it to settle for 30 minutes.
3. Introduce another large tray or baking sheet with paper bags topped with paper towel.

4. Place it near the stove.

5. Heat about 4 tablespoons of extra virgin oil after patting the eggplants dry over a medium temperature to a point of simmering.

6. Fry the eggplants in batches in the oil. Ensure not to crowd the skillet.

7. After the eggplants have turned golden brown on every side, remove and arrange them on a paper towel-lined tray to allowing draining and cooling.

8. Assemble the eggplants on a serving dish and sprinkle with 1 tablespoon of za'atar.

9. In a medium sized mixing bowl, combine the cucumbers, chickpeas, parsley, red onions, tomatoes, and the dill.

10. Add the remaining za'atar and stir gently

11. In a separate small bowl, whisk the dressing together.

12. Drizzle 2 tablespoons of the salad dressing over the already fried eggplants.

13. The remaining dressing should be poured over the chickpeas salad mix.

14. Add the chickpea salad to the eggplant in a serving dish.

15. Enjoy.

Chicken sharwarma salad bowls

Ingredients

- ¾ tablespoon of garlic powder
- Salt
- ¾ tablespoon of paprika
- ¾ tablespoon of ground coriander
- 8 boneless, skinless chicken thighs
- ¾ tablespoon of ground cumin
- ½ teaspoon of ground cloves
- ½ teaspoon of cayenne pepper
- ¾ tablespoon of turmeric powder
- ⅓ cup extra virgin olive oil
- 1 large onion, thinly sliced
- 1 large lemon, juice of
- 1 garlic clove minced
- 8 oz. baby arugula
- 2 to 3 Roma tomatoes, diced
- Sumac approximately ½ teaspoon
- Juice of 1 lemon
- Extra Virgin Olive Oil
- ¼ red onion, thinly sliced
- 1 English cucumber, diced
- Salt and pepper

Directions

1. In a small bowl, mix majority of the ingredients typically the coriander, turmeric, cumin, garlic power, paprika, and cloves.
2. Keep the sharwarma spice for later
3. Pat the chicken thighs dry and season with salt on both sides.
4. Then thinly slice into small bite-sized pieces.
5. Put the chicken in a large bowl, then add the shawarma spices, then toss to coat.
6. Introduce the onions, olive oil, and lemon juice.
7. Toss everything together to combine, then set aside as you prepare the salad
8. Cover totally for refrigeration for up to 3 hours. If there is time for you to wait, refrigerate overnight.
9. Prepare the salad in a mixing bowl by combining the tomatoes, cucumbers, arugula, and onions over a medium temperature.
10. In a separate small bowl combine the olive oil, garlic, pepper, salt, sumac, and lemon juice to make the dressing, blend thoroughly well.
11. Pour the dressing over the salad and toss to let combine.
12. Heat another extra virgin olive oil in a large skillet over medium temperature until when it simmers without smoke.
13. Add the chicken and let cook for 5 – 6 minutes.

14. Toss and continue to cook for another 5 – 6 minute until when the chicken is ready.
15. Divide the salad into serving dishes, then add the ready cooked chicken sharwarma.
16. Serve and enjoy with pit wedges if desired.

Mediterranean couscous salad

This salad recipe is yet loaded with flavorful and highly nutritious from sources such as fresh herbs, chickpeas, zippy lemon dill vinaigrette.

Other than that, the dish is famous for its versatility for lunch, supper and or breakfast. Interestingly, it can be made ahead of time before hunger hunts you down.

Ingredients

- 15-20 fresh basil leaves, roughly chopped or torn
- Water
- 1 tsp dill weed
- 15 ounces can chickpeas
- 2 cups Pearl Couscous
- salt and pepper
- Private Reserve extra virgin olive oil
- 1 large lemon, juice of
- 14 ounces can artichoke hearts
- ⅓ cup extra virgin olive oil
- ½ English cucumber, chopped
- 2 cups grape tomatoes, halved
- ½ cup pitted Kalamata olive
- ⅓ cup finely chopped red onions

- 1 to 2 garlic cloves, minced
- 3 ounces of fresh baby mozzarella optional

Directions

1. Place all the vinaigrette ingredients in a bowl to make the lemon-dill vinaigrette.
2. Whisk together to combine keep aside for a short while.
3. In a medium-sized pot, heat two tablespoons of olive oil .
4. Briefly, Sauté the couscous in the olive oil to turn golden brown.
5. Add boiling water about 3 cups or as instructed to cook the couscous.
6. Drain excess water in a colander when ready and also keep aside in a bowl allow to cool.
7. Combine all the remaining ingredients except the basil and mozzarella in a large mixing bowl.
8. Add the couscous and the basil and mix together gently
9. It is time to give the lemon-dill vinaigrette a quick whisk, also add to the couscous salad.
10. Mix again to combine.
11. Test and adjust the salt accordingly.
12. Lastly, mix in the mozzarella cheese and garnish with more fresh basil.
13. Serve and enjoy.

Mediterranean cauliflower salad

Ingredients

- Extra virgin olive oil
- 1 whole bunch of parsley, stems partially removed
- Kosher salt and pepper
- 1 English cucumber chopped
- ½ red onion, chopped
- 1 head raw cauliflower, cut into florets
- 1 to 2 garlic cloves, minced
- 3 – 4 Roma tomatoes, chopped
- Juice of 2 lemons

Directions

1. In a bowl of a food processor fitted with a blade, put the cauliflower florets.
2. Pulse briefly until the cauliflower turns rice-like in texture.
3. Move chopped cauliflower into a larger bowl.
4. Add the parsley, cucumbers, tomatoes, and onions let toss to combine.
5. Add minced garlic and season with salt and pepper.
6. Add fresh lemon juice and drizzle with extra virgin olive oil.

7. Toss once again to combine.

8. Keep the cauliflower salad aside for some minutes let soften and absorb dressing.

9. Serve and enjoy.

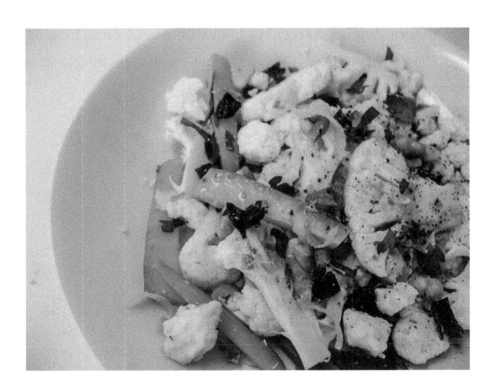

Watermelon cups

This recipe is largely and appetizer pretty and sweet to enjoy.

In addition, watermelon is a gift to the kidney which boosts its functionality.

The watermelon cut into cubes hold with a refreshing topping that shows red onions, fresh herbs and cucumber brings out a person's appetite to eat them.

Ingredients

- 15 – 17 watermelon cubes without seeds
- 5 teaspoons of red onions finely chopped
- 2 teaspoons of mint freshly minced
- 1/3 cups of chopped cucumber
- 2 teaspoons of fresh cilantro minced
- ½ teaspoon of lime juice

Directions

1. In a watermelon baller, measure spoon, scoop the watermelon blossoms form the center of the cubes.
2. Do not totally remove the center of the watermelon, leave about 1/4 in

3. Mix all the remaining ingredients in a separate small bowl
4. Spoon it into watermelon cubes
5. Serve and enjoy your watermelon cups for a healthy kidney

Simple green juice

15 minutes is all it takes to make this handful 6 ingredients healthy juice with its refreshing tast

Ingredients

- 5 celery stalks, ends trimmed
- Handful fresh parsley, 1 ounce
- 1 Inch piece of fresh peeled ginger
- 1 bunch kale, 5 ounces
- ½ large English cucumber
- 1 Granny smith apple

Directions

1. Prep all the vegetables after washing.
2. Add all the ingredients into a juicer and blend at once.
3. Pour the green juice to glasses and serve immediately.
4. Enjoy.

Mixed beery smoothie

If you do not like chopping of ingredient, then this is a perfect Mediterranean smoothie you can go for.

It gets ready in only 5 minutes.

All you need is to blend all the ingredients at once.

Ingredients

- ⅛ cup honey
- ⅓ cup Greek yogurt
- 2 ripe bananas
- 2 cups frozen mixed berry
- 1 cup milk

Directions

1. In a blender, combine bananas together with the, frozen berry mix, milk, Greek yogurt, and honey.
2. Blend until finely smooth.
3. Serve and enjoy.

Apple pear ginger smoothie

This is a dairy free recipe with variety of fruits and ginger as a flavor.

It is rich with antioxidants and vitamins from the 5 ingredients.

Ingredients

- 1½ cup of apple juice
- ½ cup rolled oats
- 1 thumb-size ginger, finely grated
- 3 pears cored and diced
- 3 apples preferably red, peeled and diced

Directions

1. Process the oats until they are powdery in a food processor.
2. Add the remaining ingredients, process until smooth
3. Serve and enjoy immediately.

Detox green juice

Among the Mediterranean Sea diet recipes, detox green juice is a perfect immunity booster and a body cleanser.

It takes 10 minutes to prepare.

Ingredients

- ½ small lemon, juice only
- 7 ounces of fresh kale
- ½ English of cucumber
- 3 large green apples
- 1 cup fresh spinach

Directions

1. Cut the apples into quarters, kale, and cucumber pieces
2. Using a juicer, juice everything else apart from the lemon.
3. Taste and adjust accordingly with lemon.
4. Serve and enjoy.

Mango kale smoothie

A combination of mango and kale (herb) makes a wonderful healthy smoothie packed with vitamins and antioxidants.

Ingredients

- 2 tablespoons of honey
- 1 medium banana, cut into chunks
- ½ cup of Greek yogurt
- 1 cup of frozen mango pieces
- 2 cups of chopped kale leaves
- 1 cup of milk

Directions

1. Combine every ingredient into a blender.
2. Blend until it becomes smooth.
3. Transfer into a glass.
4. Serve and enjoy.

Matcha iced tea

Matcha iced tea is a perfect Mediterranean Sea diet for a refreshing drink with mint and a ton of flavors.

Ingredients

- 1 lime
- 1 cup of crushed ice
- 2 teaspoon of matcha powder
- 2 cups of cold water
- 5 tablespoon of maple syrup
- 1/4 cup of hot water
- 3 sprigs of fresh mint

Directions

1. Combine and mix matcha powder in water in a small dish, mix.
2. Place in crushed ice, cold water together with fresh mint in a blender.
3. Add in the matcha tea blend briefly for 1 minute.
4. Drain.
5. Add juice and maple syrup after half of the time has run up.

6. Garnish with mint leaves and lime.

7. Serve and enjoy.

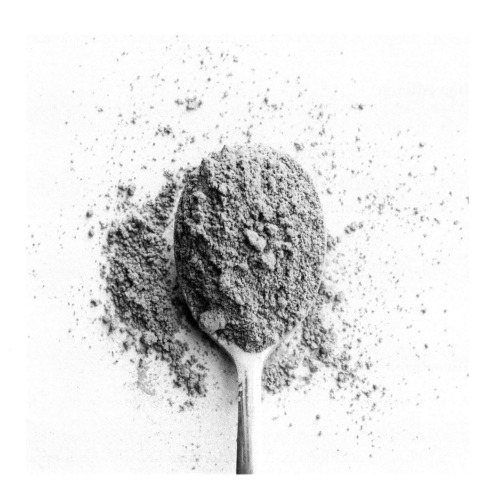

Lemon lime cucumber water

It is a perfect alternative to quenching you thirst to taking water.

It is entirely sugar free making vegetarian.

This recipe also helps to chop weight and detox the body.

Ingredients

- 4 cups Water
- 2 Limes
- 12 slices Lemon
- 16 slices Cucumber

Directions

1. Combine sliced lemon, lime, and cucumber in a jar.
2. Pour water over the jar and cover tightly.
3. Allow the water to infuse in a refrigerator for 4 hours.
4. Serve and enjoy.

Muddled mint and cucumber cooler cocktail

Ingredients

- 1 small cucumber, sliced
- 1 oz. gin
- ¼ cup of fresh mint leaves
- 1 cup of lemonade
- Ice

Directions

1. Begin by muddling 4 slices of cucumber with the mint in a shaker together with the ice, lemonade and gin.
2. Shake well and pour into a tall 8-ounce glass.
3. Garnish with extra cucumber slices and mint leaves.
4. Serve and enjoy.

Mint lemonade

Mint lemonade gives a refreshing taste to this recipe blended with lemon juice.

In 5 minutes your juice will be ready.

Ingredients

- 6 mint sprigs
- 4 cups of water
- 3 lemons
- 3 tablespoons of granulated sugar

Directions

1. Pour water in a large pitcher.
2. Add sugar and freshly squeezed juice from 2 lemons.
3. Stir to dissolved the sugar.
4. Then, add the mint sprigs together with the lemon slices.
5. Cover the pitcher with the lid.
6. Refrigerate for 2 hours.
7. Serve and enjoy.

Pineapple infused water

This is a method of replenishing the lost water in your body especially if you do not prefer to take water.

But it is recommended to take natural water anyway.

Ingredients

- 2 – 4 Sprigs Mint
- 1 Pineapple
- 4 cups Water

Directions

1. Cut the pineapple and slice thinly.
2. Dice the juicy flesh.
3. Place in a jug.
4. Add a bit of mint sprigs with water.
5. Cover well and refrigerate to let infuse overnight.
6. Strain the water and keep refrigerated.
7. Serve and enjoy.

Spinach cucumber smoothie

If you lack vitamins and antioxidants in your diet, make sure your boost them with this recipe because they are rich in these food values.

Ingredients

- 8 pitted dates
- 1 cucumber
- 1 medium apple
- 1 avocado
- 1½ cup of spinach, packed
- 2 cups almond milk

Directions

1. Peel and dice both the apple and the cucumber.
2. Cut the avocado in half, remove the seed.
3. Chop the dates roughly.
4. Combine all the ingredients in a blender.
5. Let blend until smooth.

Watermelon beet juice

Watermelon with beet is a perfect Mediterranean Sea diet fruit combination for total hydration and boosting of blood supply by the beet.

It is quite refreshing.

Ingredients

- Mint
- 2 Medium Beets
- 2.5 pounds Watermelon
- Lemon

Directions

1. Prepare the fruits by washing and peeling.
2. Place all of them in a blender.
3. Blends until every flesh is crushed into juice.
4. Taste and adjust accordingly with the lemon.
5. Garnish with mint and watermelon wedge, if you like.
6. Serve and enjoy immediately.
7. Refrigerate the balance.

Immune boosting turmeric tea

Take charge of your immunity health by making this Mediterranean magical recipe.

It blends in turmeric root, mind and ginger flavors.

Ingredients

- A pinch of black pepper , per cup
- 2 cups water
- 2 – 3 fresh mint sprigs
- 1 thumb size ginger root
- 1 orange, small
- 1 thumb size turmeric root

Directions

1. Firstly, start by boiling water.
2. Clean the turmeric, ginger, orange, and mint; peel and slice the turmeric and ginger. Cut the orange into half.
3. Divide ingredients in 2 mugs.
4. Add in boiling water over it.
5. Add a pinch of black pepper.
6. Squeeze orange juice (a little bit).
7. Allow it to steep for 15 minutes.
8. Serve and drink.

Watermelon juice with grapes

This recipe combines mint with honey, grapes and some extra flavor.

Ingredients

- 10 white grapes
- 4 cups of watermelon pieces
- Ice cubes
- 2 tablespoons of freshly squeezed lemon juice
- 3 tablespoons of honey
- 10 mint leaves

Directions

1. Cut watermelon into chunks.
2. Place in a blender along with the mint leaves and blend to combine.
3. Place into glasses together with grapes, ice cubes and garnish with mint.
4. Serve and enjoy immediately.

Orange infused water

With turmeric and citrus flavor this Mediterranean Sea diet recipe is a perfect choice to quench your thirst.

It is tasty and very refreshing.

Ingredients

- 4 cups of water
- 4 basil sprigs
- 1 large orange
- 2 turmeric roots

Directions

1. Wash and slice the orange.
2. Peel and slice turmeric roots.
3. Place water in a large jug.
4. Add the orange slices together with the turmeric and basil.
5. Cover and chill in the fridge for 12 hours.
6. Serve and enjoy.

Energy boosting smoothie with papaya and avocado

This recipe is a bomb blast of vitamin, fiber with immunity boosting properties.

The can get a sufficient energy from this Mediterranean fruity diet recipe.

Ingredients

- 2 Oranges
- 1 lb. Papaya
- 1 Banana
- 1 Avocado

Directions

1. Peel all the fruits, remove seeds and chop into chinks.
2. Place everything a food processor.
3. Squeeze orange juice in it.
4. Process until smooth.
5. Serve in your glass and enjoy immediately.

Cloudy apple pear juice

Ingredients

- 6 Apples
- 3 Pears

Directions

1. Cut apples and pears, after cleaning, into quarters and core them.
2. Juice both in a juicer.
3. Serve and enjoy.

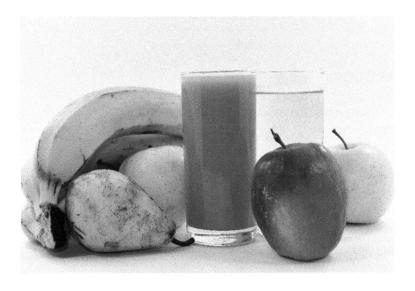

Orange Julius

Oranges are used with milk and vanillas to make this healthy and tasty juice.

You can use any sweetener to add more sweet taste if needed.

Ingredients

- 1 teaspoon of Vanilla Extract
- 1/4 cup Milk
- 6 Oranges, medium-large
- 2 tablespoons of Maple Syrup
- 1 cup Ice

Directions

1. Squeeze the juice out of the oranges.
2. Place in a blender.
3. Add ice together with milk, maple syrup, and vanilla extract.
4. Blend until smooth and creamy.
5. Serve in glasses and enjoy immediately.

Watermelon Agua Fresca

This is a sugar free recipe with low calorie content.

It is fresh and refreshing especially during summer times.

Ingredients

- 2 teaspoons of maple syrup
- 6 cups of watermelon chunks
- 5 teaspoons of fresh lemon juice
- 1 cup of water

Directions

1. In a blender, put all the ingredients except lemon juice.
2. Blend until ready.
3. Add 5 teaspoons lemon juice, stir.
4. Taste and adjust accordingly.
5. Strain, serve and enjoy.

Basic blueberry smoothie

This basic blueberry smoothie is a very luscious breakfast recipe with high nutrition content.

It is highly creamy made with frozen blueberries, almond milk and butter as well as bananas.

Ingredients

- 1/4 cup of almond butter
- 1 ½ cups of to 2 cups unsweetened vanilla almond milk or water
- 2 teaspoons of maple syrup, if necessary
- 1 ½ cups of frozen blueberries
- 1 ½ cup of frozen bananas

Directions

1. In a blender, combine all of the ingredients.
2. Blend gently and increase gradually.
3. Continue blending up to the highest blender speed.
4. Keep scarping the mixture from the sides of the blender.
5. You can add more milk at this point if you like.
6. After the smoothie is very creamy, feel free to taste.

7. You can then add the maple syrup in case you prefer a sweeter smoothie.
8. Divide the smoothie into glasses.
9. Serve immediately and enjoy.

Banana almond smoothie

This Mediterranean Sea diet recipe per harps takes the shortest time to prepare.

In 5 minutes or less, your creamy banana smooth will just be ready to quench your appetite for it.

Ingredients

- ½ cup of almond milk, yogurt
- 1 medium to large frozen banana
- Tiny drop of almond extract
- 1 heaping spoonful of almond butter
- Drizzle of honey, agave nectar
- 2 spoonfuls of flax seed

Directions

1. Toss all the ingredients into a blender at once and blend until smooth or to your liking.
2. Pour into a glass
3. Enjoy.

Roasted tomato basil soup

The roasted tomato recipe derived its delicacy power from aromatic fresh herbs especially thyme and other spices.

The use of extra virgin olive oil propels it to the next level of a wonderful finish with a heavy cream.

Ingredients

- 2 to 3 carrots peeled and cut into small chunks
- 5 garlic cloves minced
- ½ teaspoon of ground cumin
- 2 ½ cups water
- 1 teaspoon of dry oregano
- Salt and pepper
- Extra virgin olive oil
- ½ teaspoon of paprika
- 2 medium yellow onions chopped
- 1 cup canned crushed tomatoes
- 2 oz. fresh basil leaves
- 3 lb. Roma tomatoes halved
- Splash of lime juice optional
- 3 – 4 fresh thyme springs 2 tsp thyme leaves

Directions

1. Heat oven ready to 450°.
2. Combine tomatoes and carrot pieces in a large mixing bowl.
3. Drizzle the extra virgin olive oil over it, then season with kosher salt and black pepper.
4. Toss to combine.
5. Change to a large baking sheet and spread well in one layer.
6. Roast in the heated oven for 30 minutes.
7. Remove when ready from the heat and set keep aside for 10 minutes to allow cooling.
8. Move the roasted tomatoes along with the carrots to a food processor fitted with a blade.
9. Add little water for blending.
10. Heat 2 tablespoon of extra virgin olive oil over medium-high temperature until it shimmers in a large cooking pot.
11. Introduce the onions and cook for 3 minutes.
12. Introduce the garlic and cook shortly until golden.
13. Pour the roasted tomato mixture into the cooking pot.
14. Stir in the crushed tomatoes, basil, spices, thyme and ½ of water
15. Season with a little kosher salt and black pepper.
16. Boil, then reduce the heat and cover part-way to let simmer for 20 minutes.

17. Remove the thyme springs and transfer tomato basil soup to serving bowls.
18. Serve with crusty bread and enjoy.

Quinoa vegetables soup

This is purely a Mediterranean Sea diet soup feature with several variety of vegetables, herbs and quinoa.

Gluten free, it is a perfect healthy option for you.

Ingredients

- 2 celery stalks, chopped
- 6 garlic cloves, minced
- 1 large can of diced tomatoes
- 3 carrots, peeled and chopped
- 2 cups of chopped vegetables
- Scant 1 cup of quinoa, rinsed
- 4 cups of vegetable broth
- 2 cups of water
- 1 medium onion, chopped
- 1 teaspoon of salt
- 2 bay leaves
- Pinch red pepper flakes
- 3 tablespoons of extra virgin olive oil
- Ground black pepper
- 1 can of great northern beans
- 1 cup of chopped fresh kale
- 2 teaspoons of lemon juice
- ½ teaspoon of dried thyme

Directions

1. Warm olive oil in a large oven over medium heat till shimmering.
2. Add carrot, chopped onion, seasonal vegetables, celery, and a pinch of salt.
3. Let cook as you stir frequently, until onion are translucent in 6 – 8 minutes.
4. Add garlic together with thyme.
5. Cook until fragrant while stirring frequently in 1 minute.
6. Stir in the diced tomatoes cook for briefly minutes, stirring frequently.
7. Pour in the broth, quinoa, and the water.
8. Add 2 bay leaves, 1 teaspoon of salt, and a pinch of red pepper flakes.
9. Season with ground black pepper.
10. Increase the heat let boil.
11. Partially cover the pot and reduce heat to let simmer for 25 minutes.
12. Add beans along with chopped greens.
13. Simmering for 5 minutes.
14. Take off heat, remove the bay leaves.
15. Stir in 1 teaspoon lemon juice.
16. Taste and season accordingly.
17. Divide into bowls.
18. Serve and enjoy.

Mediterranean spicy spinach lentil soup

Ingredient

- 2 cups chopped flat leaf parsley
- Greek Extra Virgin Olive Oil
- 1 ½ teaspoon of sumac
- 6 cups low-sodium vegetable broth
- 1 large garlic clove, chopped
- Salt and pepper
- • 1 ½ cups green lentils or small brown lentils
- Pinch of sugar
- 1 large yellow onion, chopped
- • 1 ½ teaspoon of ground cumin
- 12 oz. frozen cut leaf spinach
- 1 ½ teaspoon of crushed red peppers
- 2 teaspoon of dried mint flakes
- 3 cups water, more if needed
- 1 ½ teaspoon of ground coriander
- 1 lime juice
- 1 tablespoon flour

Directions

1. In a large cast iron pot , heat 2 tablespoon of olive oil.

2. Add the chopped onions and continue to Sauté until turns golden brown.

3. Introduce the garlic, dried mint, flour, sugar, and all the spices and cook for 2 minutes over medium heat, keep stirring frequently.

4. Add broth and water.

5. Increase the heat to high enough to bring the liquid to a rolling boil

6. Introduce the frozen spinach and the lentils to the content.

7. On a high temperature cook for 5 minutes.

8. Lower the heat to medium cook for 20 minutes when covered.

9. When the lentils are fully cooked, stir in the lime juice and chopped parsley.

10. Remove from the heat cover and let settle for 5 minutes.

11. Serve hot with pita bread.

Simple mushroom barley soup

Seeking for a deliciously comfortable vegetable soup?

This simple mushroom soup is the perfect answer with perfect flavors and subtle smoky finish.

Ingredients

- Black pepper
- Extra virgin olive oil
- 2 celery stalks, chopped
- 1 yellow onion, chopped
- Kosher salt
- 1 cup pearl barley rinsed
- ½ - 3/4 teaspoon of smoked paprika
- 4 garlic cloves, chopped
- 8 ounces of white mushrooms, cleaned and chopped
- ½ cup canned crushed tomatoes
- 1 teaspoon of coriander
- ½ teaspoon of cumin
- 6 cups low-sodium broth
- 1 carrot, chopped
- ½ cup packed chopped parsley
- 16 ounces of baby Bella mushrooms, sliced

Directions

1. In a large oven, heat extra virgin olive oil over medium-high temperature to shimmer without smoke.
2. Add baby bell mushrooms and cook until mushrooms soften to gain some color in approximately 5 minutes thereabout.
3. Remove from the pot and keep aside.
4. Using the same pot, add small extra virgin olive oil.
5. Add onions, celery, chopped white mushrooms, and carrots, then let cook for 4 – 5 minutes over medium temperature.
6. Season with the salt and pepper.
7. Introduce the crushed tomatoes and coriander, smoked paprika, and cumin.
8. Let cook for 3 minutes, keep tossing frequently.
9. Add both the broth and pearl barley.
10. Bring to a rolling boil for 5 minutes
11. Remove the heat let simmer over low temperature for 45 minutes until tender or cooked through.
12. Transfer the cooked Bella mushrooms back to the pot and stir to blend.
13. Continue to cook for 5 minutes to warm the mushrooms through.
14. Finish with fresh parsley.
15. Serving in bowls.
16. Enjoy.

Cold cucumber soup

Ingredients

- Lemon juice
- Salt, to taste
- 2 pounds of fresh cucumbers, peeled and diced
- ¼ cup fresh parsley, chopped
- ½ cup fresh dill, chopped
- 1 cup Greek yogurt
- Black pepper
- ½ cup water
- 1 medium onion, quartered

Directions

1. In a blender, combine diced cucumbers together with the Greek yogurt, pinch of black pepper, dill, onion, chopped parsley, salt and water. Blend until smooth.
2. Taste and adjust accordingly.
3. Drizzle some lemon juice over and blend again.
4. Serve and enjoy chilled.

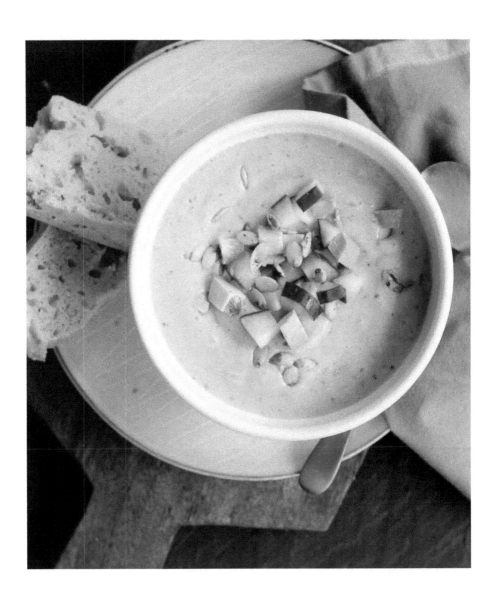